Blood Sugar
Log Book

Belongs to

_____

_____

_____

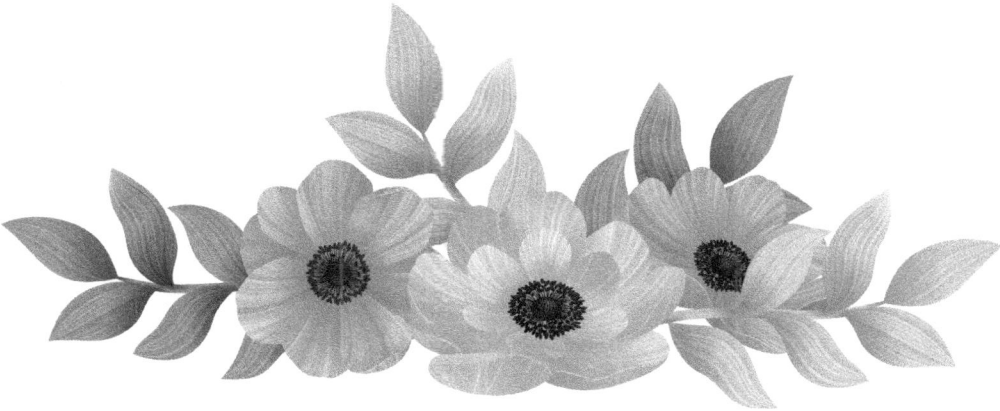

Personal Data

Name _____

Phone _____

Adress _____

In case of emergency
Please contact

Name _____

Phone _____

Adress _____

Essential Contacts

Doctor _____

Pharmacy _____

Eye Clinic _____

Dentist _____

Name _____

Cell: _____

Work: _____

Home: _____

Email: _____

Others: _____

Name _____

Cell: _____

Work: _____

Home: _____

Email: _____

Others: _____

Name _____

Cell: _____

Work: _____

Home: _____

Email: _____

Others: _____

Name _____

Cell: _____

Work: _____

Home: _____

Email: _____

Others: _____

Notes

Notes

Notes

Weekly Blood Sugar Log

Week_____

	Time	Before	After	Notes
Monday	Breakfast			
	Lunch			
	Dinner			
	Bedtime			
Tuesday	Breakfast			
	Lunch			
	Dinner			
	Bedtime			
Wednesday	Breakfast			
	Lunch			
	Dinner			
	Bedtime			
Thursday	Breakfast			
	Lunch			
	Dinner			
	Bedtime			
Friday	Breakfast			
	Lunch			
	Dinner			
	Bedtime			
Saturday	Breakfast			
	Lunch			
	Dinner			
	Bedtime			
Sunday	Breakfast			
	Lunch			
	Dinner			
	Bedtime			

Additional Notes

_____

_____

_____

_____

Weekly Blood Sugar Log

Week_____

	Time	Before	After	Notes
Monday	Breakfast			
	Lunch			
	Dinner			
	Bedtime			
Tuesday	Breakfast			
	Lunch			
	Dinner			
	Bedtime			
Wednesday	Breakfast			
	Lunch			
	Dinner			
	Bedtime			
Thursday	Breakfast			
	Lunch			
	Dinner			
	Bedtime			
Friday	Breakfast			
	Lunch			
	Dinner			
	Bedtime			
Saturday	Breakfast			
	Lunch			
	Dinner			
	Bedtime			
Sunday	Breakfast			
	Lunch			
	Dinner			
	Bedtime			

Additional Notes

_____

_____

_____

_____

Weekly Blood Sugar Log

Week_____

	Time	Before	After	Notes
Monday	Breakfast			
	Lunch			
	Dinner			
	Bedtime			
Tuesday	Breakfast			
	Lunch			
	Dinner			
	Bedtime			
Wednesday	Breakfast			
	Lunch			
	Dinner			
	Bedtime			
Thursday	Breakfast			
	Lunch			
	Dinner			
	Bedtime			
Friday	Breakfast			
	Lunch			
	Dinner			
	Bedtime			
Saturday	Breakfast			
	Lunch			
	Dinner			
	Bedtime			
Sunday	Breakfast			
	Lunch			
	Dinner			
	Bedtime			

Additional Notes

_____

_____

_____

_____

Weekly Blood Sugar Log

Week_____

	Time	Before	After	Notes
Monday	Breakfast			
	Lunch			
	Dinner			
	Bedtime			
Tuesday	Breakfast			
	Lunch			
	Dinner			
	Bedtime			
Wednesday	Breakfast			
	Lunch			
	Dinner			
	Bedtime			
Thursday	Breakfast			
	Lunch			
	Dinner			
	Bedtime			
Friday	Breakfast			
	Lunch			
	Dinner			
	Bedtime			
Saturday	Breakfast			
	Lunch			
	Dinner			
	Bedtime			
Sunday	Breakfast			
	Lunch			
	Dinner			
	Bedtime			

Additional Notes

_____

_____

_____

_____

Weekly Blood Sugar Log

Week_____

	Time	Before	After	Notes
Monday	Breakfast			
	Lunch			
	Dinner			
	Bedtime			
Tuesday	Breakfast			
	Lunch			
	Dinner			
	Bedtime			
Wednesday	Breakfast			
	Lunch			
	Dinner			
	Bedtime			
Thursday	Breakfast			
	Lunch			
	Dinner			
	Bedtime			
Friday	Breakfast			
	Lunch			
	Dinner			
	Bedtime			
Saturday	Breakfast			
	Lunch			
	Dinner			
	Bedtime			
Sunday	Breakfast			
	Lunch			
	Dinner			
	Bedtime			

Additional Notes

_____

_____

_____

_____

Weekly Blood Sugar Log

Week_____

	Time	Before	After	Notes
Monday	Breakfast			
	Lunch			
	Dinner			
	Bedtime			
Tuesday	Breakfast			
	Lunch			
	Dinner			
	Bedtime			
Wednesday	Breakfast			
	Lunch			
	Dinner			
	Bedtime			
Thursday	Breakfast			
	Lunch			
	Dinner			
	Bedtime			
Friday	Breakfast			
	Lunch			
	Dinner			
	Bedtime			
Saturday	Breakfast			
	Lunch			
	Dinner			
	Bedtime			
Sunday	Breakfast			
	Lunch			
	Dinner			
	Bedtime			

Additional Notes

_____

_____

_____

_____

Weekly Blood Sugar Log

Week_____

	Time	Before	After	Notes
Monday	Breakfast			
	Lunch			
	Dinner			
	Bedtime			
Tuesday	Breakfast			
	Lunch			
	Dinner			
	Bedtime			
Wednesday	Breakfast			
	Lunch			
	Dinner			
	Bedtime			
Thursday	Breakfast			
	Lunch			
	Dinner			
	Bedtime			
Friday	Breakfast			
	Lunch			
	Dinner			
	Bedtime			
Saturday	Breakfast			
	Lunch			
	Dinner			
	Bedtime			
Sunday	Breakfast			
	Lunch			
	Dinner			
	Bedtime			

Additional Notes

_____

_____

_____

_____

Weekly Blood Sugar Log

Week_____

	Time	Before	After	Notes
Monday	Breakfast			
	Lunch			
	Dinner			
	Bedtime			
Tuesday	Breakfast			
	Lunch			
	Dinner			
	Bedtime			
Wednesday	Breakfast			
	Lunch			
	Dinner			
	Bedtime			
Thursday	Breakfast			
	Lunch			
	Dinner			
	Bedtime			
Friday	Breakfast			
	Lunch			
	Dinner			
	Bedtime			
Saturday	Breakfast			
	Lunch			
	Dinner			
	Bedtime			
Sunday	Breakfast			
	Lunch			
	Dinner			
	Bedtime			

Additional Notes

_____

_____

_____

_____

Weekly Blood Sugar Log

Week_____

	Time	Before	After	Notes
Monday	Breakfast			
	Lunch			
	Dinner			
	Bedtime			
Tuesday	Breakfast			
	Lunch			
	Dinner			
	Bedtime			
Wednesday	Breakfast			
	Lunch			
	Dinner			
	Bedtime			
Thursday	Breakfast			
	Lunch			
	Dinner			
	Bedtime			
Friday	Breakfast			
	Lunch			
	Dinner			
	Bedtime			
Saturday	Breakfast			
	Lunch			
	Dinner			
	Bedtime			
Sunday	Breakfast			
	Lunch			
	Dinner			
	Bedtime			

Additional Notes

_____

_____

_____

_____

Weekly Blood Sugar Log

Week_____

	Time	Before	After	Notes
Monday	Breakfast			
	Lunch			
	Dinner			
	Bedtime			
Tuesday	Breakfast			
	Lunch			
	Dinner			
	Bedtime			
Wednesday	Breakfast			
	Lunch			
	Dinner			
	Bedtime			
Thursday	Breakfast			
	Lunch			
	Dinner			
	Bedtime			
Friday	Breakfast			
	Lunch			
	Dinner			
	Bedtime			
Saturday	Breakfast			
	Lunch			
	Dinner			
	Bedtime			
Sunday	Breakfast			
	Lunch			
	Dinner			
	Bedtime			

Additional Notes

_____

_____

_____

_____

Weekly Blood Sugar Log

Week_____

	Time	Before	After	Notes
Monday	Breakfast			
	Lunch			
	Dinner			
	Bedtime			
Tuesday	Breakfast			
	Lunch			
	Dinner			
	Bedtime			
Wednesday	Breakfast			
	Lunch			
	Dinner			
	Bedtime			
Thursday	Breakfast			
	Lunch			
	Dinner			
	Bedtime			
Friday	Breakfast			
	Lunch			
	Dinner			
	Bedtime			
Saturday	Breakfast			
	Lunch			
	Dinner			
	Bedtime			
Sunday	Breakfast			
	Lunch			
	Dinner			
	Bedtime			

Additional Notes

_____

_____

_____

_____

Weekly Blood Sugar Log

Week_____

	Time	Before	After	Notes
Monday	Breakfast			
	Lunch			
	Dinner			
	Bedtime			
Tuesday	Breakfast			
	Lunch			
	Dinner			
	Bedtime			
Wednesday	Breakfast			
	Lunch			
	Dinner			
	Bedtime			
Thursday	Breakfast			
	Lunch			
	Dinner			
	Bedtime			
Friday	Breakfast			
	Lunch			
	Dinner			
	Bedtime			
Saturday	Breakfast			
	Lunch			
	Dinner			
	Bedtime			
Sunday	Breakfast			
	Lunch			
	Dinner			
	Bedtime			

Additional Notes

_____

_____

_____

_____

Weekly Blood Sugar Log

Week_____

	Time	Before	After	Notes
Monday	Breakfast			
	Lunch			
	Dinner			
	Bedtime			
Tuesday	Breakfast			
	Lunch			
	Dinner			
	Bedtime			
Wednesday	Breakfast			
	Lunch			
	Dinner			
	Bedtime			
Thursday	Breakfast			
	Lunch			
	Dinner			
	Bedtime			
Friday	Breakfast			
	Lunch			
	Dinner			
	Bedtime			
Saturday	Breakfast			
	Lunch			
	Dinner			
	Bedtime			
Sunday	Breakfast			
	Lunch			
	Dinner			
	Bedtime			

Additional Notes

_____

_____

_____

_____

Weekly Blood Sugar Log

Week_____

	Time	Before	After	Notes
Monday	Breakfast			
	Lunch			
	Dinner			
	Bedtime			
Tuesday	Breakfast			
	Lunch			
	Dinner			
	Bedtime			
Wednesday	Breakfast			
	Lunch			
	Dinner			
	Bedtime			
Thursday	Breakfast			
	Lunch			
	Dinner			
	Bedtime			
Friday	Breakfast			
	Lunch			
	Dinner			
	Bedtime			
Saturday	Breakfast			
	Lunch			
	Dinner			
	Bedtime			
Sunday	Breakfast			
	Lunch			
	Dinner			
	Bedtime			

Additional Notes

_____

_____

_____

_____

Weekly Blood Sugar Log

Week_____

	Time	Before	After	Notes
Monday	Breakfast			
	Lunch			
	Dinner			
	Bedtime			
Tuesday	Breakfast			
	Lunch			
	Dinner			
	Bedtime			
Wednesday	Breakfast			
	Lunch			
	Dinner			
	Bedtime			
Thursday	Breakfast			
	Lunch			
	Dinner			
	Bedtime			
Friday	Breakfast			
	Lunch			
	Dinner			
	Bedtime			
Saturday	Breakfast			
	Lunch			
	Dinner			
	Bedtime			
Sunday	Breakfast			
	Lunch			
	Dinner			
	Bedtime			

Additional Notes

Weekly Blood Sugar Log

Week_____

	Time	Before	After	Notes
Monday	Breakfast			
	Lunch			
	Dinner			
	Bedtime			
Tuesday	Breakfast			
	Lunch			
	Dinner			
	Bedtime			
Wednesday	Breakfast			
	Lunch			
	Dinner			
	Bedtime			
Thursday	Breakfast			
	Lunch			
	Dinner			
	Bedtime			
Friday	Breakfast			
	Lunch			
	Dinner			
	Bedtime			
Saturday	Breakfast			
	Lunch			
	Dinner			
	Bedtime			
Sunday	Breakfast			
	Lunch			
	Dinner			
	Bedtime			

Additional Notes

_____

_____

_____

_____

Weekly Blood Sugar Log

Week_____

	Time	Before	After	Notes
Monday	Breakfast			
	Lunch			
	Dinner			
	Bedtime			
Tuesday	Breakfast			
	Lunch			
	Dinner			
	Bedtime			
Wednesday	Breakfast			
	Lunch			
	Dinner			
	Bedtime			
Thursday	Breakfast			
	Lunch			
	Dinner			
	Bedtime			
Friday	Breakfast			
	Lunch			
	Dinner			
	Bedtime			
Saturday	Breakfast			
	Lunch			
	Dinner			
	Bedtime			
Sunday	Breakfast			
	Lunch			
	Dinner			
	Bedtime			

Additional Notes

_____

_____

_____

_____

Weekly Blood Sugar Log

Week_____

	Time	Before	After	Notes
Monday	Breakfast			
	Lunch			
	Dinner			
	Bedtime			
Tuesday	Breakfast			
	Lunch			
	Dinner			
	Bedtime			
Wednesday	Breakfast			
	Lunch			
	Dinner			
	Bedtime			
Thursday	Breakfast			
	Lunch			
	Dinner			
	Bedtime			
Friday	Breakfast			
	Lunch			
	Dinner			
	Bedtime			
Saturday	Breakfast			
	Lunch			
	Dinner			
	Bedtime			
Sunday	Breakfast			
	Lunch			
	Dinner			
	Bedtime			

Additional Notes

_____

_____

_____

_____

Weekly Blood Sugar Log

Week_____

	Time	Before	After	Notes
Monday	Breakfast			
	Lunch			
	Dinner			
	Bedtime			
Tuesday	Breakfast			
	Lunch			
	Dinner			
	Bedtime			
Wednesday	Breakfast			
	Lunch			
	Dinner			
	Bedtime			
Thursday	Breakfast			
	Lunch			
	Dinner			
	Bedtime			
Friday	Breakfast			
	Lunch			
	Dinner			
	Bedtime			
Saturday	Breakfast			
	Lunch			
	Dinner			
	Bedtime			
Sunday	Breakfast			
	Lunch			
	Dinner			
	Bedtime			

Additional Notes

_____

_____

_____

_____

Weekly Blood Sugar Log

Week_____

	Time	Before	After	Notes
Monday	Breakfast			
	Lunch			
	Dinner			
	Bedtime			
Tuesday	Breakfast			
	Lunch			
	Dinner			
	Bedtime			
Wednesday	Breakfast			
	Lunch			
	Dinner			
	Bedtime			
Thursday	Breakfast			
	Lunch			
	Dinner			
	Bedtime			
Friday	Breakfast			
	Lunch			
	Dinner			
	Bedtime			
Saturday	Breakfast			
	Lunch			
	Dinner			
	Bedtime			
Sunday	Breakfast			
	Lunch			
	Dinner			
	Bedtime			

Additional Notes

_____

_____

_____

_____

Weekly Blood Sugar Log

Week_____

	Time	Before	After	Notes
Monday	Breakfast			
	Lunch			
	Dinner			
	Bedtime			
Tuesday	Breakfast			
	Lunch			
	Dinner			
	Bedtime			
Wednesday	Breakfast			
	Lunch			
	Dinner			
	Bedtime			
Thursday	Breakfast			
	Lunch			
	Dinner			
	Bedtime			
Friday	Breakfast			
	Lunch			
	Dinner			
	Bedtime			
Saturday	Breakfast			
	Lunch			
	Dinner			
	Bedtime			
Sunday	Breakfast			
	Lunch			
	Dinner			
	Bedtime			

Additional Notes

_____

_____

_____

_____

Weekly Blood Sugar Log

Week_____

	Time	Before	After	Notes
Monday	Breakfast			
	Lunch			
	Dinner			
	Bedtime			
Tuesday	Breakfast			
	Lunch			
	Dinner			
	Bedtime			
Wednesday	Breakfast			
	Lunch			
	Dinner			
	Bedtime			
Thursday	Breakfast			
	Lunch			
	Dinner			
	Bedtime			
Friday	Breakfast			
	Lunch			
	Dinner			
	Bedtime			
Saturday	Breakfast			
	Lunch			
	Dinner			
	Bedtime			
Sunday	Breakfast			
	Lunch			
	Dinner			
	Bedtime			

Additional Notes

_____

_____

_____

_____

Weekly Blood Sugar Log

Week_____

	Time	Before	After	Notes
Monday	Breakfast			
	Lunch			
	Dinner			
	Bedtime			
Tuesday	Breakfast			
	Lunch			
	Dinner			
	Bedtime			
Wednesday	Breakfast			
	Lunch			
	Dinner			
	Bedtime			
Thursday	Breakfast			
	Lunch			
	Dinner			
	Bedtime			
Friday	Breakfast			
	Lunch			
	Dinner			
	Bedtime			
Saturday	Breakfast			
	Lunch			
	Dinner			
	Bedtime			
Sunday	Breakfast			
	Lunch			
	Dinner			
	Bedtime			

Additional Notes

_____

_____

_____

_____

Weekly Blood Sugar Log

Week_____

	Time	Before	After	Notes
Monday	Breakfast			
	Lunch			
	Dinner			
	Bedtime			
Tuesday	Breakfast			
	Lunch			
	Dinner			
	Bedtime			
Wednesday	Breakfast			
	Lunch			
	Dinner			
	Bedtime			
Thursday	Breakfast			
	Lunch			
	Dinner			
	Bedtime			
Friday	Breakfast			
	Lunch			
	Dinner			
	Bedtime			
Saturday	Breakfast			
	Lunch			
	Dinner			
	Bedtime			
Sunday	Breakfast			
	Lunch			
	Dinner			
	Bedtime			

Additional Notes

_____

_____

_____

_____

Weekly Blood Sugar Log

Week_____

	Time	Before	After	Notes
Monday	Breakfast			
	Lunch			
	Dinner			
	Bedtime			
Tuesday	Breakfast			
	Lunch			
	Dinner			
	Bedtime			
Wednesday	Breakfast			
	Lunch			
	Dinner			
	Bedtime			
Thursday	Breakfast			
	Lunch			
	Dinner			
	Bedtime			
Friday	Breakfast			
	Lunch			
	Dinner			
	Bedtime			
Saturday	Breakfast			
	Lunch			
	Dinner			
	Bedtime			
Sunday	Breakfast			
	Lunch			
	Dinner			
	Bedtime			

Additional Notes

_____

_____

_____

_____

Weekly Blood Sugar Log

Week_____

	Time	Before	After	Notes
Monday	Breakfast			
	Lunch			
	Dinner			
	Bedtime			
Tuesday	Breakfast			
	Lunch			
	Dinner			
	Bedtime			
Wednesday	Breakfast			
	Lunch			
	Dinner			
	Bedtime			
Thursday	Breakfast			
	Lunch			
	Dinner			
	Bedtime			
Friday	Breakfast			
	Lunch			
	Dinner			
	Bedtime			
Saturday	Breakfast			
	Lunch			
	Dinner			
	Bedtime			
Sunday	Breakfast			
	Lunch			
	Dinner			
	Bedtime			

Additional Notes

_____

_____

_____

_____

Weekly Blood Sugar Log

Week_____

	Time	Before	After	Notes
Monday	Breakfast			
	Lunch			
	Dinner			
	Bedtime			
Tuesday	Breakfast			
	Lunch			
	Dinner			
	Bedtime			
Wednesday	Breakfast			
	Lunch			
	Dinner			
	Bedtime			
Thursday	Breakfast			
	Lunch			
	Dinner			
	Bedtime			
Friday	Breakfast			
	Lunch			
	Dinner			
	Bedtime			
Saturday	Breakfast			
	Lunch			
	Dinner			
	Bedtime			
Sunday	Breakfast			
	Lunch			
	Dinner			
	Bedtime			

Additional Notes

_____

_____

_____

_____

Weekly Blood Sugar Log

Week_____

	Time	Before	After	Notes
Monday	Breakfast			
	Lunch			
	Dinner			
	Bedtime			
Tuesday	Breakfast			
	Lunch			
	Dinner			
	Bedtime			
Wednesday	Breakfast			
	Lunch			
	Dinner			
	Bedtime			
Thursday	Breakfast			
	Lunch			
	Dinner			
	Bedtime			
Friday	Breakfast			
	Lunch			
	Dinner			
	Bedtime			
Saturday	Breakfast			
	Lunch			
	Dinner			
	Bedtime			
Sunday	Breakfast			
	Lunch			
	Dinner			
	Bedtime			

Additional Notes

_____

_____

_____

_____

Weekly Blood Sugar Log

Week_____

	Time	Before	After	Notes
Monday	Breakfast			
	Lunch			
	Dinner			
	Bedtime			
Tuesday	Breakfast			
	Lunch			
	Dinner			
	Bedtime			
Wednesday	Breakfast			
	Lunch			
	Dinner			
	Bedtime			
Thursday	Breakfast			
	Lunch			
	Dinner			
	Bedtime			
Friday	Breakfast			
	Lunch			
	Dinner			
	Bedtime			
Saturday	Breakfast			
	Lunch			
	Dinner			
	Bedtime			
Sunday	Breakfast			
	Lunch			
	Dinner			
	Bedtime			

Additional Notes

_____

_____

_____

_____

Weekly Blood Sugar Log

Week_____

	Time	Before	After	Notes
Monday	Breakfast			
	Lunch			
	Dinner			
	Bedtime			
Tuesday	Breakfast			
	Lunch			
	Dinner			
	Bedtime			
Wednesday	Breakfast			
	Lunch			
	Dinner			
	Bedtime			
Thursday	Breakfast			
	Lunch			
	Dinner			
	Bedtime			
Friday	Breakfast			
	Lunch			
	Dinner			
	Bedtime			
Saturday	Breakfast			
	Lunch			
	Dinner			
	Bedtime			
Sunday	Breakfast			
	Lunch			
	Dinner			
	Bedtime			

Additional Notes

_____

_____

_____

_____

Weekly Blood Sugar Log

Week_____

	Time	Before	After	Notes
Monday	Breakfast			
	Lunch			
	Dinner			
	Bedtime			
Tuesday	Breakfast			
	Lunch			
	Dinner			
	Bedtime			
Wednesday	Breakfast			
	Lunch			
	Dinner			
	Bedtime			
Thursday	Breakfast			
	Lunch			
	Dinner			
	Bedtime			
Friday	Breakfast			
	Lunch			
	Dinner			
	Bedtime			
Saturday	Breakfast			
	Lunch			
	Dinner			
	Bedtime			
Sunday	Breakfast			
	Lunch			
	Dinner			
	Bedtime			

Additional Notes

_____

_____

_____

_____

Weekly Blood Sugar Log

Week_____

	Time	Before	After	Notes
Monday	Breakfast			
	Lunch			
	Dinner			
	Bedtime			
Tuesday	Breakfast			
	Lunch			
	Dinner			
	Bedtime			
Wednesday	Breakfast			
	Lunch			
	Dinner			
	Bedtime			
Thursday	Breakfast			
	Lunch			
	Dinner			
	Bedtime			
Friday	Breakfast			
	Lunch			
	Dinner			
	Bedtime			
Saturday	Breakfast			
	Lunch			
	Dinner			
	Bedtime			
Sunday	Breakfast			
	Lunch			
	Dinner			
	Bedtime			

Additional Notes

_____

_____

_____

_____

Weekly Blood Sugar Log

Week_____

	Time	Before	After	Notes
Monday	Breakfast			
	Lunch			
	Dinner			
	Bedtime			
Tuesday	Breakfast			
	Lunch			
	Dinner			
	Bedtime			
Wednesday	Breakfast			
	Lunch			
	Dinner			
	Bedtime			
Thursday	Breakfast			
	Lunch			
	Dinner			
	Bedtime			
Friday	Breakfast			
	Lunch			
	Dinner			
	Bedtime			
Saturday	Breakfast			
	Lunch			
	Dinner			
	Bedtime			
Sunday	Breakfast			
	Lunch			
	Dinner			
	Bedtime			

Additional Notes

_____

_____

_____

_____

Weekly Blood Sugar Log

Week_____

	Time	Before	After	Notes
Monday	Breakfast			
	Lunch			
	Dinner			
	Bedtime			
Tuesday	Breakfast			
	Lunch			
	Dinner			
	Bedtime			
Wednesday	Breakfast			
	Lunch			
	Dinner			
	Bedtime			
Thursday	Breakfast			
	Lunch			
	Dinner			
	Bedtime			
Friday	Breakfast			
	Lunch			
	Dinner			
	Bedtime			
Saturday	Breakfast			
	Lunch			
	Dinner			
	Bedtime			
Sunday	Breakfast			
	Lunch			
	Dinner			
	Bedtime			

Additional Notes

_____

_____

_____

_____

Weekly Blood Sugar Log

Week_____

	Time	Before	After	Notes
Monday	Breakfast			
	Lunch			
	Dinner			
	Bedtime			
Tuesday	Breakfast			
	Lunch			
	Dinner			
	Bedtime			
Wednesday	Breakfast			
	Lunch			
	Dinner			
	Bedtime			
Thursday	Breakfast			
	Lunch			
	Dinner			
	Bedtime			
Friday	Breakfast			
	Lunch			
	Dinner			
	Bedtime			
Saturday	Breakfast			
	Lunch			
	Dinner			
	Bedtime			
Sunday	Breakfast			
	Lunch			
	Dinner			
	Bedtime			

Additional Notes

_____

_____

_____

_____

Weekly Blood Sugar Log

Week_____

	Time	Before	After	Notes
Monday	Breakfast			
	Lunch			
	Dinner			
	Bedtime			
Tuesday	Breakfast			
	Lunch			
	Dinner			
	Bedtime			
Wednesday	Breakfast			
	Lunch			
	Dinner			
	Bedtime			
Thursday	Breakfast			
	Lunch			
	Dinner			
	Bedtime			
Friday	Breakfast			
	Lunch			
	Dinner			
	Bedtime			
Saturday	Breakfast			
	Lunch			
	Dinner			
	Bedtime			
Sunday	Breakfast			
	Lunch			
	Dinner			
	Bedtime			

Additional Notes

_____

_____

_____

_____

Weekly Blood Sugar Log

Week_____

	Time	Before	After	Notes
Monday	Breakfast			
	Lunch			
	Dinner			
	Bedtime			
Tuesday	Breakfast			
	Lunch			
	Dinner			
	Bedtime			
Wednesday	Breakfast			
	Lunch			
	Dinner			
	Bedtime			
Thursday	Breakfast			
	Lunch			
	Dinner			
	Bedtime			
Friday	Breakfast			
	Lunch			
	Dinner			
	Bedtime			
Saturday	Breakfast			
	Lunch			
	Dinner			
	Bedtime			
Sunday	Breakfast			
	Lunch			
	Dinner			
	Bedtime			

Additional Notes

_____

_____

_____

_____

Weekly Blood Sugar Log

Week_____

	Time	Before	After	Notes
Monday	Breakfast			
	Lunch			
	Dinner			
	Bedtime			
Tuesday	Breakfast			
	Lunch			
	Dinner			
	Bedtime			
Wednesday	Breakfast			
	Lunch			
	Dinner			
	Bedtime			
Thursday	Breakfast			
	Lunch			
	Dinner			
	Bedtime			
Friday	Breakfast			
	Lunch			
	Dinner			
	Bedtime			
Saturday	Breakfast			
	Lunch			
	Dinner			
	Bedtime			
Sunday	Breakfast			
	Lunch			
	Dinner			
	Bedtime			

Additional Notes

_____

_____

_____

_____

Weekly Blood Sugar Log

Week_____

	Time	Before	After	Notes
Monday	Breakfast			
	Lunch			
	Dinner			
	Bedtime			
Tuesday	Breakfast			
	Lunch			
	Dinner			
	Bedtime			
Wednesday	Breakfast			
	Lunch			
	Dinner			
	Bedtime			
Thursday	Breakfast			
	Lunch			
	Dinner			
	Bedtime			
Friday	Breakfast			
	Lunch			
	Dinner			
	Bedtime			
Saturday	Breakfast			
	Lunch			
	Dinner			
	Bedtime			
Sunday	Breakfast			
	Lunch			
	Dinner			
	Bedtime			

Additional Notes

_____

_____

_____

_____

Weekly Blood Sugar Log

Week_____

	Time	Before	After	Notes
Monday	Breakfast			
	Lunch			
	Dinner			
	Bedtime			
Tuesday	Breakfast			
	Lunch			
	Dinner			
	Bedtime			
Wednesday	Breakfast			
	Lunch			
	Dinner			
	Bedtime			
Thursday	Breakfast			
	Lunch			
	Dinner			
	Bedtime			
Friday	Breakfast			
	Lunch			
	Dinner			
	Bedtime			
Saturday	Breakfast			
	Lunch			
	Dinner			
	Bedtime			
Sunday	Breakfast			
	Lunch			
	Dinner			
	Bedtime			

Additional Notes

_____

_____

_____

_____

Weekly Blood Sugar Log

Week_____

	Time	Before	After	Notes
Monday	Breakfast			
	Lunch			
	Dinner			
	Bedtime			
Tuesday	Breakfast			
	Lunch			
	Dinner			
	Bedtime			
Wednesday	Breakfast			
	Lunch			
	Dinner			
	Bedtime			
Thursday	Breakfast			
	Lunch			
	Dinner			
	Bedtime			
Friday	Breakfast			
	Lunch			
	Dinner			
	Bedtime			
Saturday	Breakfast			
	Lunch			
	Dinner			
	Bedtime			
Sunday	Breakfast			
	Lunch			
	Dinner			
	Bedtime			

Additional Notes

_____

_____

_____

_____

Weekly Blood Sugar Log

Week_____

	Time	Before	After	Notes
Monday	Breakfast			
	Lunch			
	Dinner			
	Bedtime			
Tuesday	Breakfast			
	Lunch			
	Dinner			
	Bedtime			
Wednesday	Breakfast			
	Lunch			
	Dinner			
	Bedtime			
Thursday	Breakfast			
	Lunch			
	Dinner			
	Bedtime			
Friday	Breakfast			
	Lunch			
	Dinner			
	Bedtime			
Saturday	Breakfast			
	Lunch			
	Dinner			
	Bedtime			
Sunday	Breakfast			
	Lunch			
	Dinner			
	Bedtime			

Additional Notes

_____

_____

_____

_____

Weekly Blood Sugar Log

Week_____

	Time	Before	After	Notes
Monday	Breakfast			
	Lunch			
	Dinner			
	Bedtime			
Tuesday	Breakfast			
	Lunch			
	Dinner			
	Bedtime			
Wednesday	Breakfast			
	Lunch			
	Dinner			
	Bedtime			
Thursday	Breakfast			
	Lunch			
	Dinner			
	Bedtime			
Friday	Breakfast			
	Lunch			
	Dinner			
	Bedtime			
Saturday	Breakfast			
	Lunch			
	Dinner			
	Bedtime			
Sunday	Breakfast			
	Lunch			
	Dinner			
	Bedtime			

Additional Notes

_____

_____

_____

_____

Weekly Blood Sugar Log

Week_____

	Time	Before	After	Notes
Monday	Breakfast			
	Lunch			
	Dinner			
	Bedtime			
Tuesday	Breakfast			
	Lunch			
	Dinner			
	Bedtime			
Wednesday	Breakfast			
	Lunch			
	Dinner			
	Bedtime			
Thursday	Breakfast			
	Lunch			
	Dinner			
	Bedtime			
Friday	Breakfast			
	Lunch			
	Dinner			
	Bedtime			
Saturday	Breakfast			
	Lunch			
	Dinner			
	Bedtime			
Sunday	Breakfast			
	Lunch			
	Dinner			
	Bedtime			

Additional Notes

_____

_____

_____

_____

Weekly Blood Sugar Log

Week_____

	Time	Before	After	Notes
Monday	Breakfast			
	Lunch			
	Dinner			
	Bedtime			
Tuesday	Breakfast			
	Lunch			
	Dinner			
	Bedtime			
Wednesday	Breakfast			
	Lunch			
	Dinner			
	Bedtime			
Thursday	Breakfast			
	Lunch			
	Dinner			
	Bedtime			
Friday	Breakfast			
	Lunch			
	Dinner			
	Bedtime			
Saturday	Breakfast			
	Lunch			
	Dinner			
	Bedtime			
Sunday	Breakfast			
	Lunch			
	Dinner			
	Bedtime			

Additional Notes

_____

_____

_____

_____

Weekly Blood Sugar Log

Week_____

	Time	Before	After	Notes
Monday	Breakfast			
	Lunch			
	Dinner			
	Bedtime			
Tuesday	Breakfast			
	Lunch			
	Dinner			
	Bedtime			
Wednesday	Breakfast			
	Lunch			
	Dinner			
	Bedtime			
Thursday	Breakfast			
	Lunch			
	Dinner			
	Bedtime			
Friday	Breakfast			
	Lunch			
	Dinner			
	Bedtime			
Saturday	Breakfast			
	Lunch			
	Dinner			
	Bedtime			
Sunday	Breakfast			
	Lunch			
	Dinner			
	Bedtime			

Additional Notes

_____

_____

_____

_____

Weekly Blood Sugar Log

Week_____

	Time	Before	After	Notes
Monday	Breakfast			
	Lunch			
	Dinner			
	Bedtime			
Tuesday	Breakfast			
	Lunch			
	Dinner			
	Bedtime			
Wednesday	Breakfast			
	Lunch			
	Dinner			
	Bedtime			
Thursday	Breakfast			
	Lunch			
	Dinner			
	Bedtime			
Friday	Breakfast			
	Lunch			
	Dinner			
	Bedtime			
Saturday	Breakfast			
	Lunch			
	Dinner			
	Bedtime			
Sunday	Breakfast			
	Lunch			
	Dinner			
	Bedtime			

Additional Notes

_____

_____

_____

_____

Weekly Blood Sugar Log

Week_____

	Time	Before	After	Notes
Monday	Breakfast			
	Lunch			
	Dinner			
	Bedtime			
Tuesday	Breakfast			
	Lunch			
	Dinner			
	Bedtime			
Wednesday	Breakfast			
	Lunch			
	Dinner			
	Bedtime			
Thursday	Breakfast			
	Lunch			
	Dinner			
	Bedtime			
Friday	Breakfast			
	Lunch			
	Dinner			
	Bedtime			
Saturday	Breakfast			
	Lunch			
	Dinner			
	Bedtime			
Sunday	Breakfast			
	Lunch			
	Dinner			
	Bedtime			

Additional Notes

_____

_____

_____

_____

Weekly Blood Sugar Log

Week_____

	Time	Before	After	Notes
Monday	Breakfast			
	Lunch			
	Dinner			
	Bedtime			
Tuesday	Breakfast			
	Lunch			
	Dinner			
	Bedtime			
Wednesday	Breakfast			
	Lunch			
	Dinner			
	Bedtime			
Thursday	Breakfast			
	Lunch			
	Dinner			
	Bedtime			
Friday	Breakfast			
	Lunch			
	Dinner			
	Bedtime			
Saturday	Breakfast			
	Lunch			
	Dinner			
	Bedtime			
Sunday	Breakfast			
	Lunch			
	Dinner			
	Bedtime			

Additional Notes

_____

_____

_____

_____

Weekly Blood Sugar Log

Week_____

	Time	Before	After	Notes
Monday	Breakfast			
	Lunch			
	Dinner			
	Bedtime			
Tuesday	Breakfast			
	Lunch			
	Dinner			
	Bedtime			
Wednesday	Breakfast			
	Lunch			
	Dinner			
	Bedtime			
Thursday	Breakfast			
	Lunch			
	Dinner			
	Bedtime			
Friday	Breakfast			
	Lunch			
	Dinner			
	Bedtime			
Saturday	Breakfast			
	Lunch			
	Dinner			
	Bedtime			
Sunday	Breakfast			
	Lunch			
	Dinner			
	Bedtime			

Additional Notes

_____

_____

_____

_____

Weekly Blood Sugar Log

Week_____

	Time	Before	After	Notes
Monday	Breakfast			
	Lunch			
	Dinner			
	Bedtime			
Tuesday	Breakfast			
	Lunch			
	Dinner			
	Bedtime			
Wednesday	Breakfast			
	Lunch			
	Dinner			
	Bedtime			
Thursday	Breakfast			
	Lunch			
	Dinner			
	Bedtime			
Friday	Breakfast			
	Lunch			
	Dinner			
	Bedtime			
Saturday	Breakfast			
	Lunch			
	Dinner			
	Bedtime			
Sunday	Breakfast			
	Lunch			
	Dinner			
	Bedtime			

Additional Notes

_____

_____

_____

_____

Weekly Blood Sugar Log

Week_____

	Time	Before	After	Notes
Monday	Breakfast			
	Lunch			
	Dinner			
	Bedtime			
Tuesday	Breakfast			
	Lunch			
	Dinner			
	Bedtime			
Wednesday	Breakfast			
	Lunch			
	Dinner			
	Bedtime			
Thursday	Breakfast			
	Lunch			
	Dinner			
	Bedtime			
Friday	Breakfast			
	Lunch			
	Dinner			
	Bedtime			
Saturday	Breakfast			
	Lunch			
	Dinner			
	Bedtime			
Sunday	Breakfast			
	Lunch			
	Dinner			
	Bedtime			

Additional Notes

_____

_____

_____

_____

Weekly Blood Sugar Log

Week_____

	Time	Before	After	Notes
Monday	Breakfast			
	Lunch			
	Dinner			
	Bedtime			
Tuesday	Breakfast			
	Lunch			
	Dinner			
	Bedtime			
Wednesday	Breakfast			
	Lunch			
	Dinner			
	Bedtime			
Thursday	Breakfast			
	Lunch			
	Dinner			
	Bedtime			
Friday	Breakfast			
	Lunch			
	Dinner			
	Bedtime			
Saturday	Breakfast			
	Lunch			
	Dinner			
	Bedtime			
Sunday	Breakfast			
	Lunch			
	Dinner			
	Bedtime			

Additional Notes

_____

_____

_____

_____

Weekly Blood Sugar Log

Week_____

	Time	Before	After	Notes
Monday	Breakfast			
	Lunch			
	Dinner			
	Bedtime			
Tuesday	Breakfast			
	Lunch			
	Dinner			
	Bedtime			
Wednesday	Breakfast			
	Lunch			
	Dinner			
	Bedtime			
Thursday	Breakfast			
	Lunch			
	Dinner			
	Bedtime			
Friday	Breakfast			
	Lunch			
	Dinner			
	Bedtime			
Saturday	Breakfast			
	Lunch			
	Dinner			
	Bedtime			
Sunday	Breakfast			
	Lunch			
	Dinner			
	Bedtime			

Additional Notes

_____

_____

_____

_____

Weekly Blood Sugar Log

Week_____

	Time	Before	After	Notes
Monday	Breakfast			
	Lunch			
	Dinner			
	Bedtime			
Tuesday	Breakfast			
	Lunch			
	Dinner			
	Bedtime			
Wednesday	Breakfast			
	Lunch			
	Dinner			
	Bedtime			
Thursday	Breakfast			
	Lunch			
	Dinner			
	Bedtime			
Friday	Breakfast			
	Lunch			
	Dinner			
	Bedtime			
Saturday	Breakfast			
	Lunch			
	Dinner			
	Bedtime			
Sunday	Breakfast			
	Lunch			
	Dinner			
	Bedtime			

Additional Notes

_____

_____

_____

_____

Weekly Blood Sugar Log

Week_____

	Time	Before	After	Notes
Monday	Breakfast			
	Lunch			
	Dinner			
	Bedtime			
Tuesday	Breakfast			
	Lunch			
	Dinner			
	Bedtime			
Wednesday	Breakfast			
	Lunch			
	Dinner			
	Bedtime			
Thursday	Breakfast			
	Lunch			
	Dinner			
	Bedtime			
Friday	Breakfast			
	Lunch			
	Dinner			
	Bedtime			
Saturday	Breakfast			
	Lunch			
	Dinner			
	Bedtime			
Sunday	Breakfast			
	Lunch			
	Dinner			
	Bedtime			

Additional Notes

_____

_____

_____

_____

Weekly Blood Sugar Log

Week_____

	Time	Before	After	Notes
Monday	Breakfast			
	Lunch			
	Dinner			
	Bedtime			
Tuesday	Breakfast			
	Lunch			
	Dinner			
	Bedtime			
Wednesday	Breakfast			
	Lunch			
	Dinner			
	Bedtime			
Thursday	Breakfast			
	Lunch			
	Dinner			
	Bedtime			
Friday	Breakfast			
	Lunch			
	Dinner			
	Bedtime			
Saturday	Breakfast			
	Lunch			
	Dinner			
	Bedtime			
Sunday	Breakfast			
	Lunch			
	Dinner			
	Bedtime			

Additional Notes

_____

_____

_____

_____

Weekly Blood Sugar Log

Week_____

	Time	Before	After	Notes
Monday	Breakfast			
	Lunch			
	Dinner			
	Bedtime			
Tuesday	Breakfast			
	Lunch			
	Dinner			
	Bedtime			
Wednesday	Breakfast			
	Lunch			
	Dinner			
	Bedtime			
Thursday	Breakfast			
	Lunch			
	Dinner			
	Bedtime			
Friday	Breakfast			
	Lunch			
	Dinner			
	Bedtime			
Saturday	Breakfast			
	Lunch			
	Dinner			
	Bedtime			
Sunday	Breakfast			
	Lunch			
	Dinner			
	Bedtime			

Additional Notes

_____

_____

_____

_____

Weekly Blood Sugar Log

Week_____

	Time	Before	After	Notes
Monday	Breakfast			
	Lunch			
	Dinner			
	Bedtime			
Tuesday	Breakfast			
	Lunch			
	Dinner			
	Bedtime			
Wednesday	Breakfast			
	Lunch			
	Dinner			
	Bedtime			
Thursday	Breakfast			
	Lunch			
	Dinner			
	Bedtime			
Friday	Breakfast			
	Lunch			
	Dinner			
	Bedtime			
Saturday	Breakfast			
	Lunch			
	Dinner			
	Bedtime			
Sunday	Breakfast			
	Lunch			
	Dinner			
	Bedtime			

Additional Notes

_____

_____

_____

_____

Weekly Blood Sugar Log

Week_____

	Time	Before	After	Notes
Monday	Breakfast			
	Lunch			
	Dinner			
	Bedtime			
Tuesday	Breakfast			
	Lunch			
	Dinner			
	Bedtime			
Wednesday	Breakfast			
	Lunch			
	Dinner			
	Bedtime			
Thursday	Breakfast			
	Lunch			
	Dinner			
	Bedtime			
Friday	Breakfast			
	Lunch			
	Dinner			
	Bedtime			
Saturday	Breakfast			
	Lunch			
	Dinner			
	Bedtime			
Sunday	Breakfast			
	Lunch			
	Dinner			
	Bedtime			

Additional Notes

_____

_____

_____

_____

Weekly Blood Sugar Log

Week_____

	Time	Before	After	Notes
Monday	Breakfast			
	Lunch			
	Dinner			
	Bedtime			
Tuesday	Breakfast			
	Lunch			
	Dinner			
	Bedtime			
Wednesday	Breakfast			
	Lunch			
	Dinner			
	Bedtime			
Thursday	Breakfast			
	Lunch			
	Dinner			
	Bedtime			
Friday	Breakfast			
	Lunch			
	Dinner			
	Bedtime			
Saturday	Breakfast			
	Lunch			
	Dinner			
	Bedtime			
Sunday	Breakfast			
	Lunch			
	Dinner			
	Bedtime			

Additional Notes

_____

_____

_____

_____

Weekly Blood Sugar Log

Week_____

	Time	Before	After	Notes
Monday	Breakfast			
	Lunch			
	Dinner			
	Bedtime			
Tuesday	Breakfast			
	Lunch			
	Dinner			
	Bedtime			
Wednesday	Breakfast			
	Lunch			
	Dinner			
	Bedtime			
Thursday	Breakfast			
	Lunch			
	Dinner			
	Bedtime			
Friday	Breakfast			
	Lunch			
	Dinner			
	Bedtime			
Saturday	Breakfast			
	Lunch			
	Dinner			
	Bedtime			
Sunday	Breakfast			
	Lunch			
	Dinner			
	Bedtime			

Additional Notes

_____

_____

_____

_____

Weekly Blood Sugar Log

Week_____

	Time	Before	After	Notes
Monday	Breakfast			
	Lunch			
	Dinner			
	Bedtime			
Tuesday	Breakfast			
	Lunch			
	Dinner			
	Bedtime			
Wednesday	Breakfast			
	Lunch			
	Dinner			
	Bedtime			
Thursday	Breakfast			
	Lunch			
	Dinner			
	Bedtime			
Friday	Breakfast			
	Lunch			
	Dinner			
	Bedtime			
Saturday	Breakfast			
	Lunch			
	Dinner			
	Bedtime			
Sunday	Breakfast			
	Lunch			
	Dinner			
	Bedtime			

Additional Notes

_____

_____

_____

_____

Weekly Blood Sugar Log

Week_____

	Time	Before	After	Notes
Monday	Breakfast			
	Lunch			
	Dinner			
	Bedtime			
Tuesday	Breakfast			
	Lunch			
	Dinner			
	Bedtime			
Wednesday	Breakfast			
	Lunch			
	Dinner			
	Bedtime			
Thursday	Breakfast			
	Lunch			
	Dinner			
	Bedtime			
Friday	Breakfast			
	Lunch			
	Dinner			
	Bedtime			
Saturday	Breakfast			
	Lunch			
	Dinner			
	Bedtime			
Sunday	Breakfast			
	Lunch			
	Dinner			
	Bedtime			

Additional Notes

_____

_____

_____

_____

Weekly Blood Sugar Log

Week_____

	Time	Before	After	Notes
Monday	Breakfast			
	Lunch			
	Dinner			
	Bedtime			
Tuesday	Breakfast			
	Lunch			
	Dinner			
	Bedtime			
Wednesday	Breakfast			
	Lunch			
	Dinner			
	Bedtime			
Thursday	Breakfast			
	Lunch			
	Dinner			
	Bedtime			
Friday	Breakfast			
	Lunch			
	Dinner			
	Bedtime			
Saturday	Breakfast			
	Lunch			
	Dinner			
	Bedtime			
Sunday	Breakfast			
	Lunch			
	Dinner			
	Bedtime			

Additional Notes

_____

_____

_____

_____

Weekly Blood Sugar Log

Week_____

	Time	Before	After	Notes
Monday	Breakfast			
	Lunch			
	Dinner			
	Bedtime			
Tuesday	Breakfast			
	Lunch			
	Dinner			
	Bedtime			
Wednesday	Breakfast			
	Lunch			
	Dinner			
	Bedtime			
Thursday	Breakfast			
	Lunch			
	Dinner			
	Bedtime			
Friday	Breakfast			
	Lunch			
	Dinner			
	Bedtime			
Saturday	Breakfast			
	Lunch			
	Dinner			
	Bedtime			
Sunday	Breakfast			
	Lunch			
	Dinner			
	Bedtime			

Additional Notes

_____

_____

_____

_____

Weekly Blood Sugar Log

Week_____

	Time	Before	After	Notes
Monday	Breakfast			
	Lunch			
	Dinner			
	Bedtime			
Tuesday	Breakfast			
	Lunch			
	Dinner			
	Bedtime			
Wednesday	Breakfast			
	Lunch			
	Dinner			
	Bedtime			
Thursday	Breakfast			
	Lunch			
	Dinner			
	Bedtime			
Friday	Breakfast			
	Lunch			
	Dinner			
	Bedtime			
Saturday	Breakfast			
	Lunch			
	Dinner			
	Bedtime			
Sunday	Breakfast			
	Lunch			
	Dinner			
	Bedtime			

Additional Notes

_____

_____

_____

_____

Weekly Blood Sugar Log

Week_____

	Time	Before	After	Notes
Monday	Breakfast			
	Lunch			
	Dinner			
	Bedtime			
Tuesday	Breakfast			
	Lunch			
	Dinner			
	Bedtime			
Wednesday	Breakfast			
	Lunch			
	Dinner			
	Bedtime			
Thursday	Breakfast			
	Lunch			
	Dinner			
	Bedtime			
Friday	Breakfast			
	Lunch			
	Dinner			
	Bedtime			
Saturday	Breakfast			
	Lunch			
	Dinner			
	Bedtime			
Sunday	Breakfast			
	Lunch			
	Dinner			
	Bedtime			

Additional Notes

_____

_____

_____

_____

Weekly Blood Sugar Log

Week_____

	Time	Before	After	Notes
Monday	Breakfast			
	Lunch			
	Dinner			
	Bedtime			
Tuesday	Breakfast			
	Lunch			
	Dinner			
	Bedtime			
Wednesday	Breakfast			
	Lunch			
	Dinner			
	Bedtime			
Thursday	Breakfast			
	Lunch			
	Dinner			
	Bedtime			
Friday	Breakfast			
	Lunch			
	Dinner			
	Bedtime			
Saturday	Breakfast			
	Lunch			
	Dinner			
	Bedtime			
Sunday	Breakfast			
	Lunch			
	Dinner			
	Bedtime			

Additional Notes

_____

_____

_____

_____

Weekly Blood Sugar Log

Week_____

	Time	Before	After	Notes
Monday	Breakfast			
	Lunch			
	Dinner			
	Bedtime			
Tuesday	Breakfast			
	Lunch			
	Dinner			
	Bedtime			
Wednesday	Breakfast			
	Lunch			
	Dinner			
	Bedtime			
Thursday	Breakfast			
	Lunch			
	Dinner			
	Bedtime			
Friday	Breakfast			
	Lunch			
	Dinner			
	Bedtime			
Saturday	Breakfast			
	Lunch			
	Dinner			
	Bedtime			
Sunday	Breakfast			
	Lunch			
	Dinner			
	Bedtime			

Additional Notes

_____

_____

_____

_____

Weekly Blood Sugar Log

Week_____

	Time	Before	After	Notes
Monday	Breakfast			
	Lunch			
	Dinner			
	Bedtime			
Tuesday	Breakfast			
	Lunch			
	Dinner			
	Bedtime			
Wednesday	Breakfast			
	Lunch			
	Dinner			
	Bedtime			
Thursday	Breakfast			
	Lunch			
	Dinner			
	Bedtime			
Friday	Breakfast			
	Lunch			
	Dinner			
	Bedtime			
Saturday	Breakfast			
	Lunch			
	Dinner			
	Bedtime			
Sunday	Breakfast			
	Lunch			
	Dinner			
	Bedtime			

Additional Notes

_____

_____

_____

_____

Weekly Blood Sugar Log

Week_____

	Time	Before	After	Notes
Monday	Breakfast			
	Lunch			
	Dinner			
	Bedtime			
Tuesday	Breakfast			
	Lunch			
	Dinner			
	Bedtime			
Wednesday	Breakfast			
	Lunch			
	Dinner			
	Bedtime			
Thursday	Breakfast			
	Lunch			
	Dinner			
	Bedtime			
Friday	Breakfast			
	Lunch			
	Dinner			
	Bedtime			
Saturday	Breakfast			
	Lunch			
	Dinner			
	Bedtime			
Sunday	Breakfast			
	Lunch			
	Dinner			
	Bedtime			

Additional Notes

_____

_____

_____

_____

Weekly Blood Sugar Log

Week_____

	Time	Before	After	Notes
Monday	Breakfast			
	Lunch			
	Dinner			
	Bedtime			
Tuesday	Breakfast			
	Lunch			
	Dinner			
	Bedtime			
Wednesday	Breakfast			
	Lunch			
	Dinner			
	Bedtime			
Thursday	Breakfast			
	Lunch			
	Dinner			
	Bedtime			
Friday	Breakfast			
	Lunch			
	Dinner			
	Bedtime			
Saturday	Breakfast			
	Lunch			
	Dinner			
	Bedtime			
Sunday	Breakfast			
	Lunch			
	Dinner			
	Bedtime			

Additional Notes

_____

_____

_____

_____

Weekly Blood Sugar Log

Week_____

	Time	Before	After	Notes
Monday	Breakfast			
	Lunch			
	Dinner			
	Bedtime			
Tuesday	Breakfast			
	Lunch			
	Dinner			
	Bedtime			
Wednesday	Breakfast			
	Lunch			
	Dinner			
	Bedtime			
Thursday	Breakfast			
	Lunch			
	Dinner			
	Bedtime			
Friday	Breakfast			
	Lunch			
	Dinner			
	Bedtime			
Saturday	Breakfast			
	Lunch			
	Dinner			
	Bedtime			
Sunday	Breakfast			
	Lunch			
	Dinner			
	Bedtime			

Additional Notes

_____

_____

_____

_____

Weekly Blood Sugar Log

Week_____

	Time	Before	After	Notes
Monday	Breakfast			
	Lunch			
	Dinner			
	Bedtime			
Tuesday	Breakfast			
	Lunch			
	Dinner			
	Bedtime			
Wednesday	Breakfast			
	Lunch			
	Dinner			
	Bedtime			
Thursday	Breakfast			
	Lunch			
	Dinner			
	Bedtime			
Friday	Breakfast			
	Lunch			
	Dinner			
	Bedtime			
Saturday	Breakfast			
	Lunch			
	Dinner			
	Bedtime			
Sunday	Breakfast			
	Lunch			
	Dinner			
	Bedtime			

Additional Notes

_____

_____

_____

_____

Weekly Blood Sugar Log

Week_____

	Time	Before	After	Notes
Monday	Breakfast			
	Lunch			
	Dinner			
	Bedtime			
Tuesday	Breakfast			
	Lunch			
	Dinner			
	Bedtime			
Wednesday	Breakfast			
	Lunch			
	Dinner			
	Bedtime			
Thursday	Breakfast			
	Lunch			
	Dinner			
	Bedtime			
Friday	Breakfast			
	Lunch			
	Dinner			
	Bedtime			
Saturday	Breakfast			
	Lunch			
	Dinner			
	Bedtime			
Sunday	Breakfast			
	Lunch			
	Dinner			
	Bedtime			

Additional Notes

_____

_____

_____

_____

Weekly Blood Sugar Log

Week_____

	Time	Before	After	Notes
Monday	Breakfast			
	Lunch			
	Dinner			
	Bedtime			
Tuesday	Breakfast			
	Lunch			
	Dinner			
	Bedtime			
Wednesday	Breakfast			
	Lunch			
	Dinner			
	Bedtime			
Thursday	Breakfast			
	Lunch			
	Dinner			
	Bedtime			
Friday	Breakfast			
	Lunch			
	Dinner			
	Bedtime			
Saturday	Breakfast			
	Lunch			
	Dinner			
	Bedtime			
Sunday	Breakfast			
	Lunch			
	Dinner			
	Bedtime			

Additional Notes

_____

_____

_____

_____

Weekly Blood Sugar Log

Week_____

	Time	Before	After	Notes
Monday	Breakfast			
	Lunch			
	Dinner			
	Bedtime			
Tuesday	Breakfast			
	Lunch			
	Dinner			
	Bedtime			
Wednesday	Breakfast			
	Lunch			
	Dinner			
	Bedtime			
Thursday	Breakfast			
	Lunch			
	Dinner			
	Bedtime			
Friday	Breakfast			
	Lunch			
	Dinner			
	Bedtime			
Saturday	Breakfast			
	Lunch			
	Dinner			
	Bedtime			
Sunday	Breakfast			
	Lunch			
	Dinner			
	Bedtime			

Additional Notes

_____

_____

_____

_____

Weekly Blood Sugar Log

Week_____

	Time	Before	After	Notes
Monday	Breakfast			
	Lunch			
	Dinner			
	Bedtime			
Tuesday	Breakfast			
	Lunch			
	Dinner			
	Bedtime			
Wednesday	Breakfast			
	Lunch			
	Dinner			
	Bedtime			
Thursday	Breakfast			
	Lunch			
	Dinner			
	Bedtime			
Friday	Breakfast			
	Lunch			
	Dinner			
	Bedtime			
Saturday	Breakfast			
	Lunch			
	Dinner			
	Bedtime			
Sunday	Breakfast			
	Lunch			
	Dinner			
	Bedtime			

Additional Notes

_____

_____

_____

_____

Weekly Blood Sugar Log

Week_____

	Time	Before	After	Notes
Monday	Breakfast			
	Lunch			
	Dinner			
	Bedtime			
Tuesday	Breakfast			
	Lunch			
	Dinner			
	Bedtime			
Wednesday	Breakfast			
	Lunch			
	Dinner			
	Bedtime			
Thursday	Breakfast			
	Lunch			
	Dinner			
	Bedtime			
Friday	Breakfast			
	Lunch			
	Dinner			
	Bedtime			
Saturday	Breakfast			
	Lunch			
	Dinner			
	Bedtime			
Sunday	Breakfast			
	Lunch			
	Dinner			
	Bedtime			

Additional Notes

_____

_____

_____

_____

Weekly Blood Sugar Log

Week_____

	Time	Before	After	Notes
Monday	Breakfast			
	Lunch			
	Dinner			
	Bedtime			
Tuesday	Breakfast			
	Lunch			
	Dinner			
	Bedtime			
Wednesday	Breakfast			
	Lunch			
	Dinner			
	Bedtime			
Thursday	Breakfast			
	Lunch			
	Dinner			
	Bedtime			
Friday	Breakfast			
	Lunch			
	Dinner			
	Bedtime			
Saturday	Breakfast			
	Lunch			
	Dinner			
	Bedtime			
Sunday	Breakfast			
	Lunch			
	Dinner			
	Bedtime			

Additional Notes

_____

_____

_____

_____

Weekly Blood Sugar Log

Week_____

	Time	Before	After	Notes
Monday	Breakfast			
	Lunch			
	Dinner			
	Bedtime			
Tuesday	Breakfast			
	Lunch			
	Dinner			
	Bedtime			
Wednesday	Breakfast			
	Lunch			
	Dinner			
	Bedtime			
Thursday	Breakfast			
	Lunch			
	Dinner			
	Bedtime			
Friday	Breakfast			
	Lunch			
	Dinner			
	Bedtime			
Saturday	Breakfast			
	Lunch			
	Dinner			
	Bedtime			
Sunday	Breakfast			
	Lunch			
	Dinner			
	Bedtime			

Additional Notes

_____

_____

_____

_____

Weekly Blood Sugar Log

Week_____

	Time	Before	After	Notes
Monday	Breakfast			
	Lunch			
	Dinner			
	Bedtime			
Tuesday	Breakfast			
	Lunch			
	Dinner			
	Bedtime			
Wednesday	Breakfast			
	Lunch			
	Dinner			
	Bedtime			
Thursday	Breakfast			
	Lunch			
	Dinner			
	Bedtime			
Friday	Breakfast			
	Lunch			
	Dinner			
	Bedtime			
Saturday	Breakfast			
	Lunch			
	Dinner			
	Bedtime			
Sunday	Breakfast			
	Lunch			
	Dinner			
	Bedtime			

Additional Notes

_____

_____

_____

_____

Weekly Blood Sugar Log

Week_____

	Time	Before	After	Notes
Monday	Breakfast			
	Lunch			
	Dinner			
	Bedtime			
Tuesday	Breakfast			
	Lunch			
	Dinner			
	Bedtime			
Wednesday	Breakfast			
	Lunch			
	Dinner			
	Bedtime			
Thursday	Breakfast			
	Lunch			
	Dinner			
	Bedtime			
Friday	Breakfast			
	Lunch			
	Dinner			
	Bedtime			
Saturday	Breakfast			
	Lunch			
	Dinner			
	Bedtime			
Sunday	Breakfast			
	Lunch			
	Dinner			
	Bedtime			

Additional Notes

_____

_____

_____

_____

Weekly Blood Sugar Log

Week_____

	Time	Before	After	Notes
Monday	Breakfast			
	Lunch			
	Dinner			
	Bedtime			
Tuesday	Breakfast			
	Lunch			
	Dinner			
	Bedtime			
Wednesday	Breakfast			
	Lunch			
	Dinner			
	Bedtime			
Thursday	Breakfast			
	Lunch			
	Dinner			
	Bedtime			
Friday	Breakfast			
	Lunch			
	Dinner			
	Bedtime			
Saturday	Breakfast			
	Lunch			
	Dinner			
	Bedtime			
Sunday	Breakfast			
	Lunch			
	Dinner			
	Bedtime			

Additional Notes

_____

_____

_____

_____

Weekly Blood Sugar Log

Week_____

	Time	Before	After	Notes
Monday	Breakfast			
	Lunch			
	Dinner			
	Bedtime			
Tuesday	Breakfast			
	Lunch			
	Dinner			
	Bedtime			
Wednesday	Breakfast			
	Lunch			
	Dinner			
	Bedtime			
Thursday	Breakfast			
	Lunch			
	Dinner			
	Bedtime			
Friday	Breakfast			
	Lunch			
	Dinner			
	Bedtime			
Saturday	Breakfast			
	Lunch			
	Dinner			
	Bedtime			
Sunday	Breakfast			
	Lunch			
	Dinner			
	Bedtime			

Additional Notes

_____

_____

_____

_____

Weekly Blood Sugar Log

Week_____

	Time	Before	After	Notes
Monday	Breakfast			
	Lunch			
	Dinner			
	Bedtime			
Tuesday	Breakfast			
	Lunch			
	Dinner			
	Bedtime			
Wednesday	Breakfast			
	Lunch			
	Dinner			
	Bedtime			
Thursday	Breakfast			
	Lunch			
	Dinner			
	Bedtime			
Friday	Breakfast			
	Lunch			
	Dinner			
	Bedtime			
Saturday	Breakfast			
	Lunch			
	Dinner			
	Bedtime			
Sunday	Breakfast			
	Lunch			
	Dinner			
	Bedtime			

Additional Notes

_____

_____

_____

_____

Weekly Blood Sugar Log

Week_____

	Time	Before	After	Notes
Monday	Breakfast			
	Lunch			
	Dinner			
	Bedtime			
Tuesday	Breakfast			
	Lunch			
	Dinner			
	Bedtime			
Wednesday	Breakfast			
	Lunch			
	Dinner			
	Bedtime			
Thursday	Breakfast			
	Lunch			
	Dinner			
	Bedtime			
Friday	Breakfast			
	Lunch			
	Dinner			
	Bedtime			
Saturday	Breakfast			
	Lunch			
	Dinner			
	Bedtime			
Sunday	Breakfast			
	Lunch			
	Dinner			
	Bedtime			

Additional Notes

_____

_____

_____

_____

Weekly Blood Sugar Log

Week_____

	Time	Before	After	Notes
Monday	Breakfast			
	Lunch			
	Dinner			
	Bedtime			
Tuesday	Breakfast			
	Lunch			
	Dinner			
	Bedtime			
Wednesday	Breakfast			
	Lunch			
	Dinner			
	Bedtime			
Thursday	Breakfast			
	Lunch			
	Dinner			
	Bedtime			
Friday	Breakfast			
	Lunch			
	Dinner			
	Bedtime			
Saturday	Breakfast			
	Lunch			
	Dinner			
	Bedtime			
Sunday	Breakfast			
	Lunch			
	Dinner			
	Bedtime			

Additional Notes

_____

_____

_____

_____

Weekly Blood Sugar Log

Week_____

	Time	Before	After	Notes
Monday	Breakfast			
	Lunch			
	Dinner			
	Bedtime			
Tuesday	Breakfast			
	Lunch			
	Dinner			
	Bedtime			
Wednesday	Breakfast			
	Lunch			
	Dinner			
	Bedtime			
Thursday	Breakfast			
	Lunch			
	Dinner			
	Bedtime			
Friday	Breakfast			
	Lunch			
	Dinner			
	Bedtime			
Saturday	Breakfast			
	Lunch			
	Dinner			
	Bedtime			
Sunday	Breakfast			
	Lunch			
	Dinner			
	Bedtime			

Additional Notes

_____

_____

_____

_____

Thank you!

WE ARE GLAD THAT YOU PURCHASED OUR BOOK!
PLEASE LET US KNOW HOW WE CAN IMPROVE IT!
YOUR FEEDBACK IS ESSENTIAL TO US.

Contact us at:

M log'Sin@gmail.com

JUST TITLE THE EMAIL 'CREATIVE' AND WE WILL

GIVE YOU SOME EXTRA SURPRISES!

CPSIA information can be obtained
at www.ICGtesting.com
Printed in the USA
LVHW062357030123
736050LV00007B/416

9 781803 852003